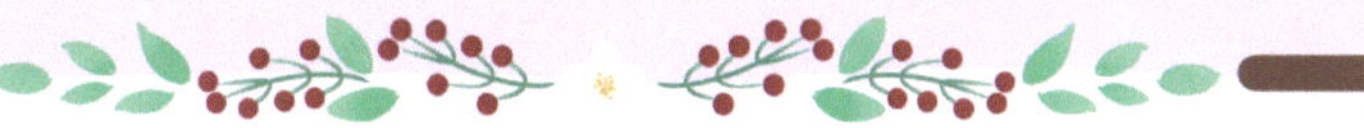

The Girl With The "Café-au-Lait" Spots

Sonia Y Meléndez & Jamaly

NF NF NF NF NF NF NF NF NF NF NF NF NF NF NF NF NF NF NF NF

Disclaimer. The content available in this book is for informational and educational purposes only and is not a substitute for the professional judgment of a health care professional in diagnosing and treating NF patients. The shared information is not intended to be used by the reader for any diagnostic purpose and are not a substitute for professional medical advice. Always seek the advice of a physician or other qualified health provider with any questions you may have regarding a medical condition.

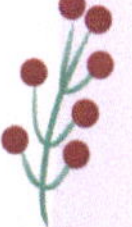

Author's information

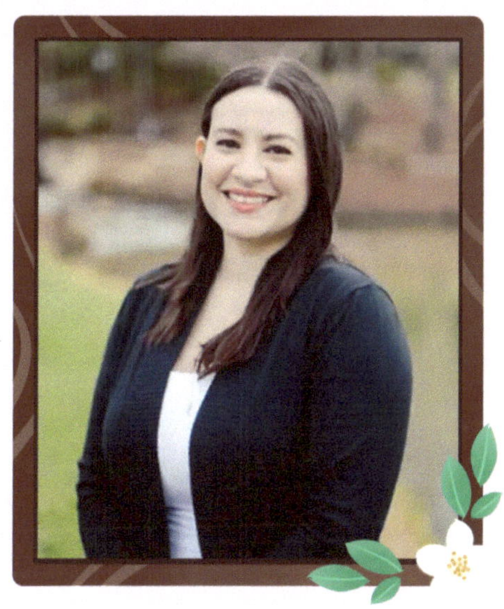

Hi, my name is Sonia Melendez, a mom who loves her daughter unconditionally. I wrote this book with the purpose of sharing what I have learned as I have walked the path of neurofibromatosis with my daughter, Jamaly/Jamy. Hope this information will help many parents understand NF; therefore, feel comfortable enough to explain it to their children.

Definitions of words identified with an *asterisk can be found on page 22 and 23. This will help you have a better understanding of NF as you read.

To Jamalyvett (Jamaly/Jamy).
You are a beautiful soul that I am blessed to call my
daughter. You are my inspiration and reason to be.

Jamy is a young NF fighter who has gone through so
much in her short life. She has been in very delicate
life/death situations in multiple occasions, but
she always comes through victorious and never stops
smiling.

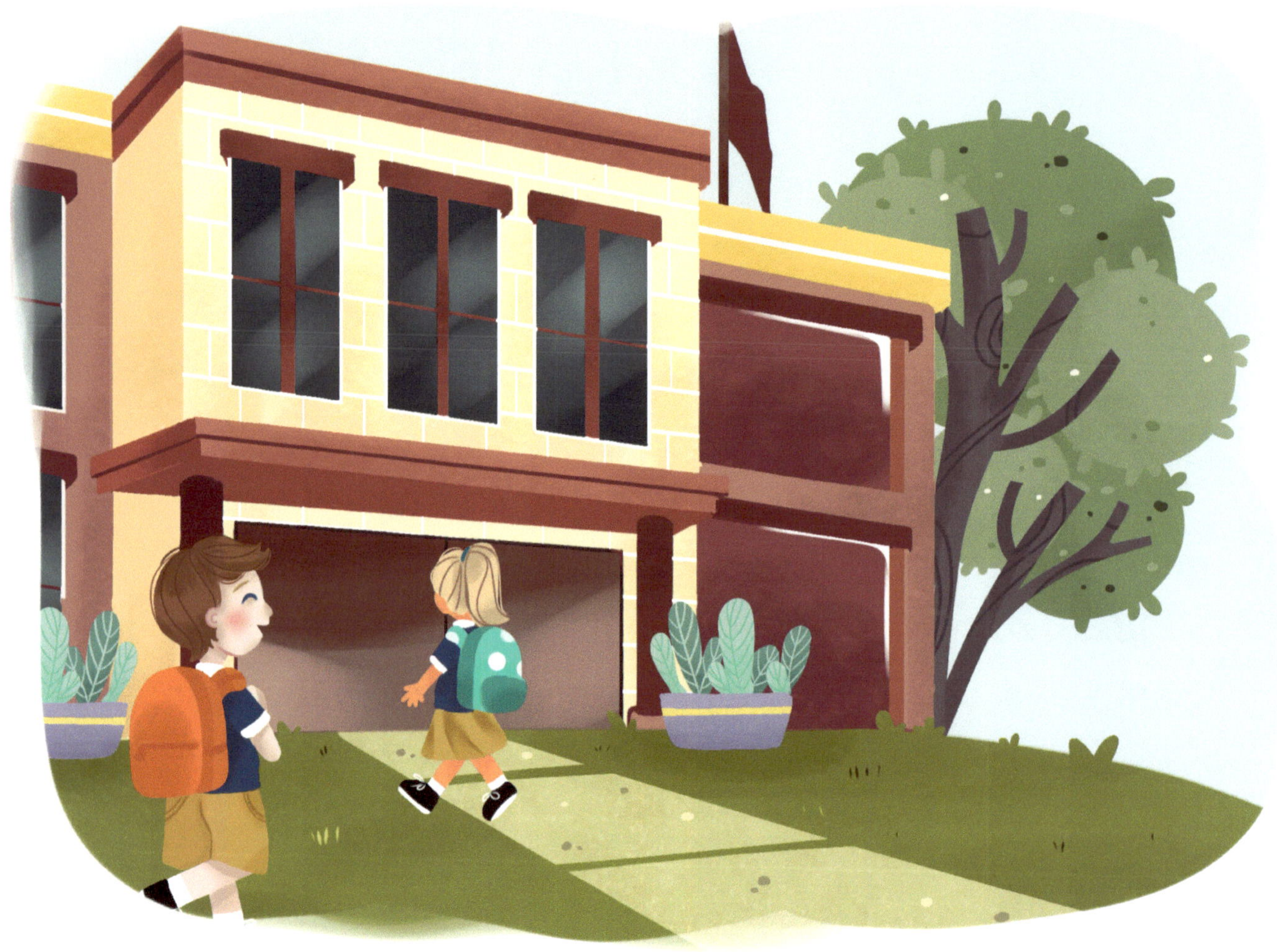

Hi my name is Jamy. I am a 6 year old girl who was born with a "genetic condition known as *Neurofibromatosis, where *tumors grow in the *nervous system. That's a big word, I know, and it's a little bit hard to say. But I can help you with that! Clap along and say it out loud with me: *Neu-ro-fi-bro-ma-to-sis.

6.

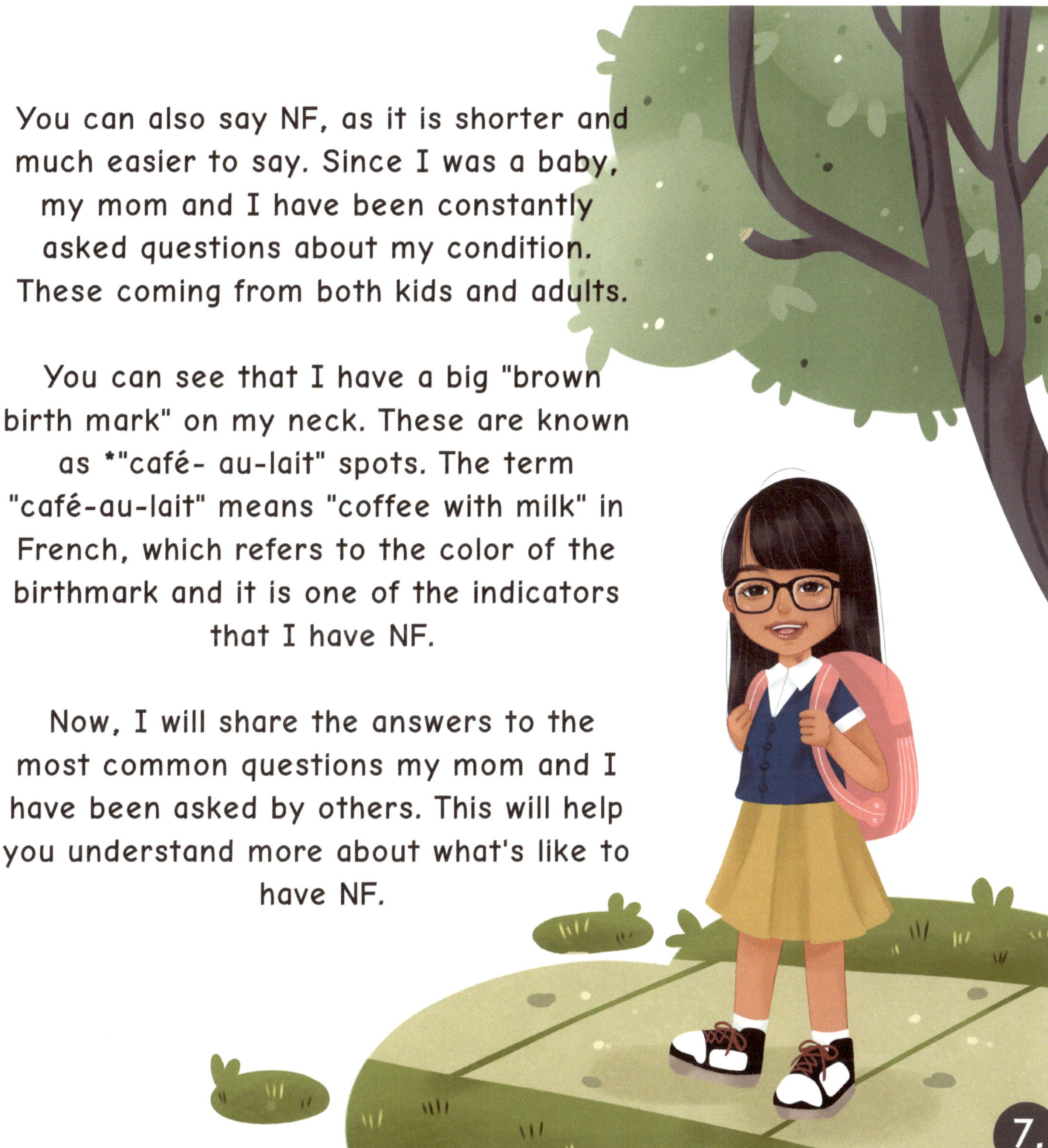

You can also say NF, as it is shorter and much easier to say. Since I was a baby, my mom and I have been constantly asked questions about my condition. These coming from both kids and adults.

You can see that I have a big "brown birth mark" on my neck. These are known as *"café- au-lait" spots. The term "café-au-lait" means "coffee with milk" in French, which refers to the color of the birthmark and it is one of the indicators that I have NF.

Now, I will share the answers to the most common questions my mom and I have been asked by others. This will help you understand more about what's like to have NF.

Why do you have NF?

In my case, as in many others it was a
*spontaneous mutation that occurred
as I was developing in my mom's belly.
In other people's cases, they may
have *inherited it from their parents,
and there's nothing they could have
done to prevent it. It is very important
to know that NF is not *contagious.

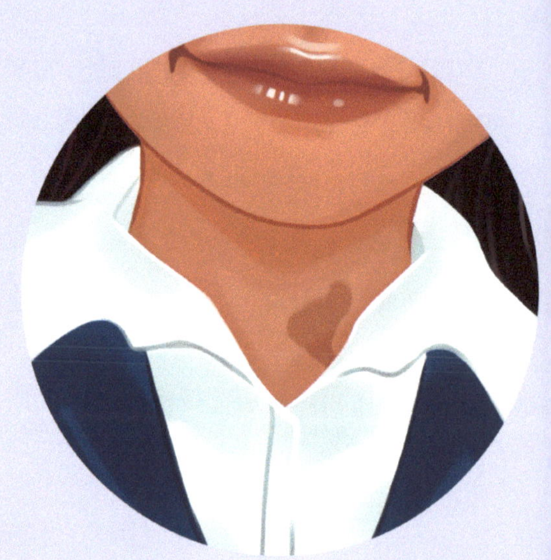

Do the tumors/neurofibromas hurt?

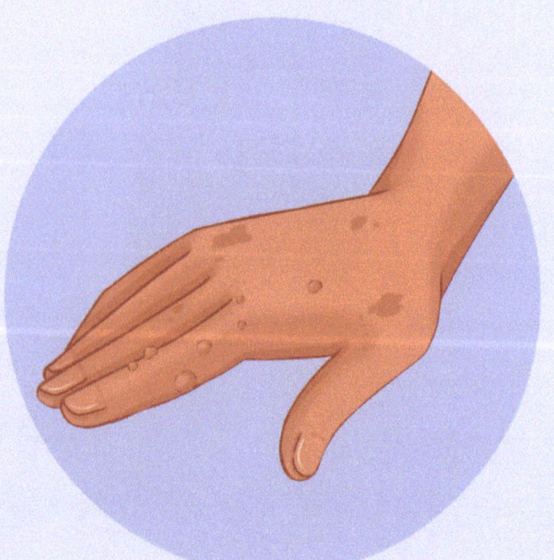

Well, it depends on where they appear.
Some might appear on my skin and
others inside my skin or organs. In most
cases, they may cause my skin to itch
and if they appear in an uncomfortable
area they could possibly hurt or bother
me. Each case is unique, and some NF
patients may never present any of these
indicators.

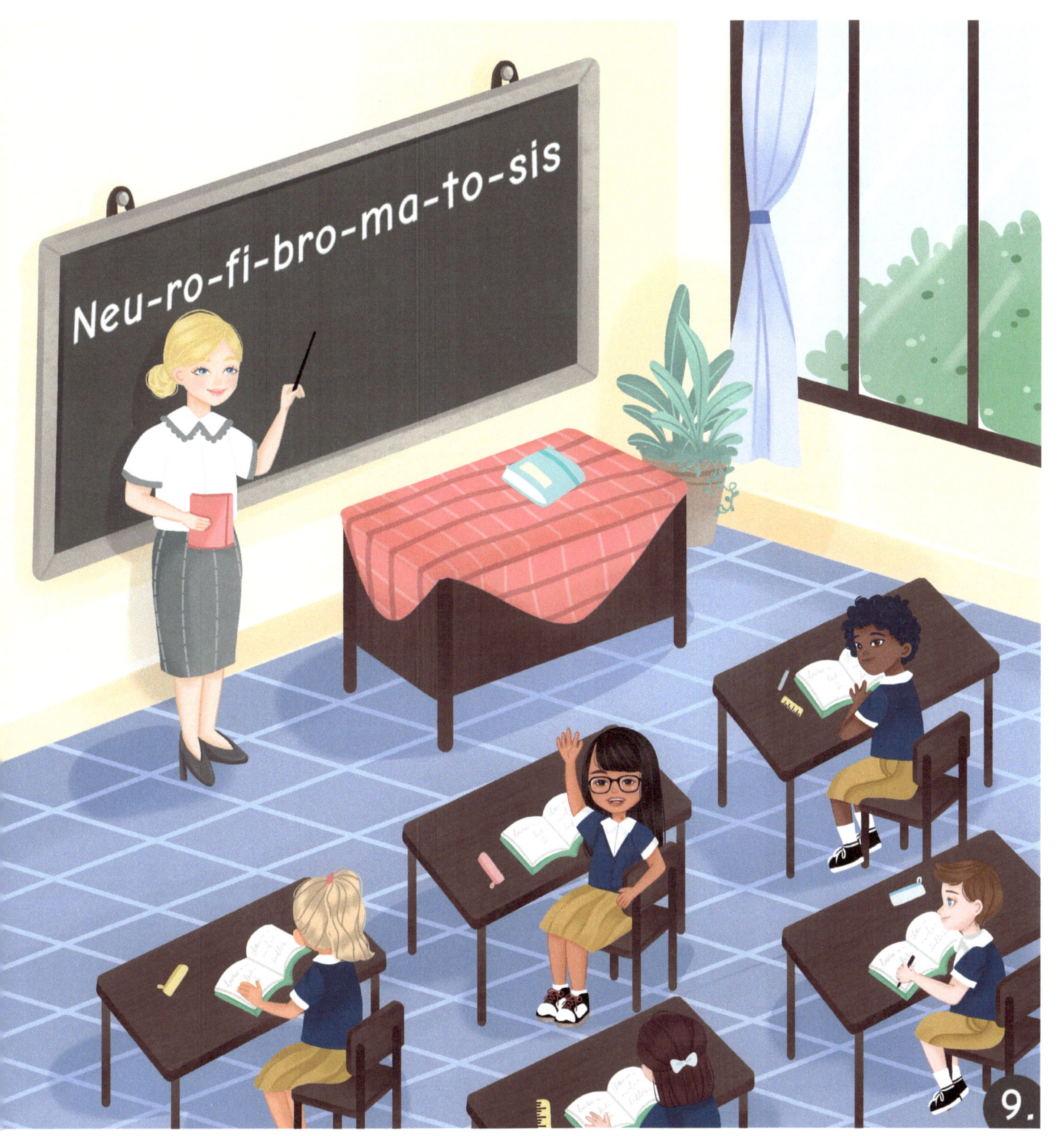
Neu-ro-fi-bro-ma-to-sis
9.

Why do you speak funny?

Well, that's because (NF) can sometimes cause for someone, like me, to have muscle weakness (*Hypotonia). When we speak, we use about 100 muscles that are all trying to work together to help us communicate and make the right sounds. But don't worry! If you can't understand me, please, just ask me to repeat myself. I will always appreciate your patience!

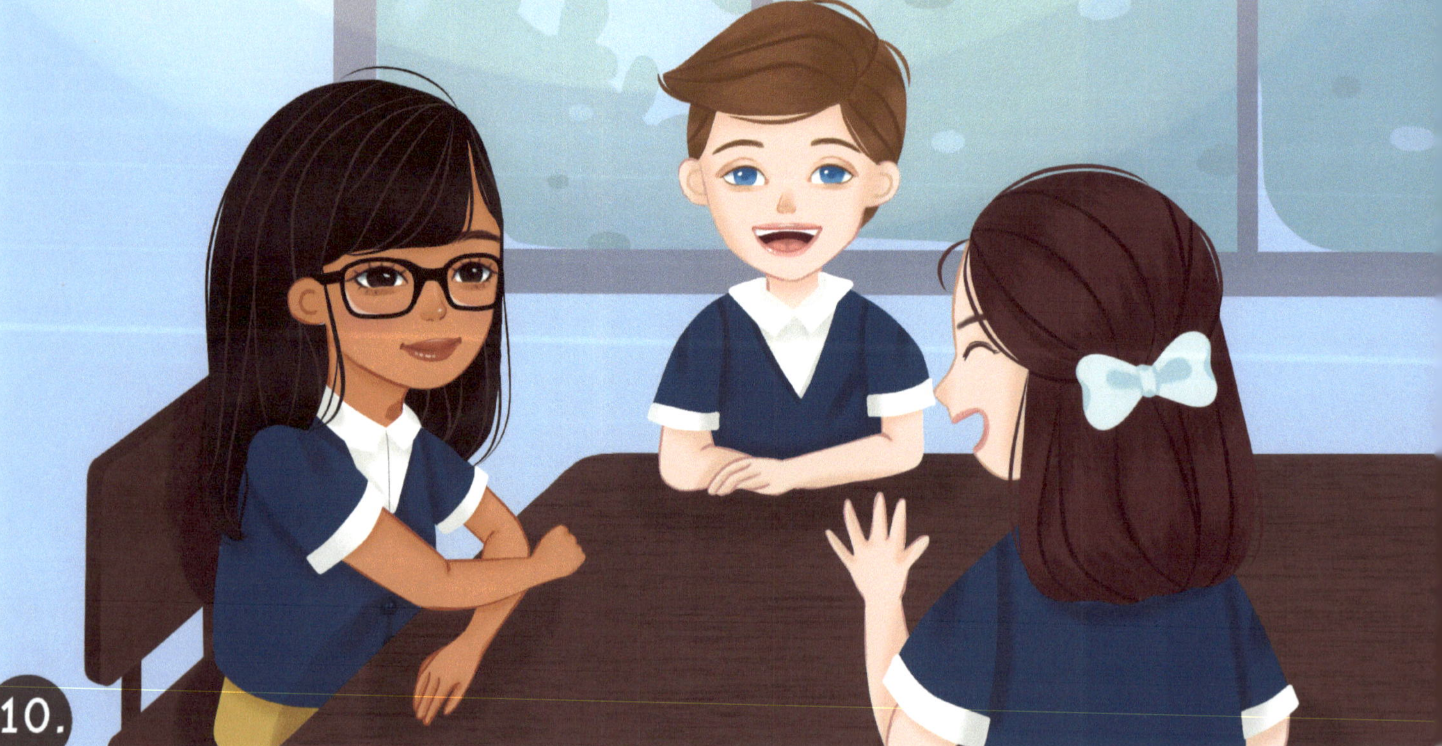

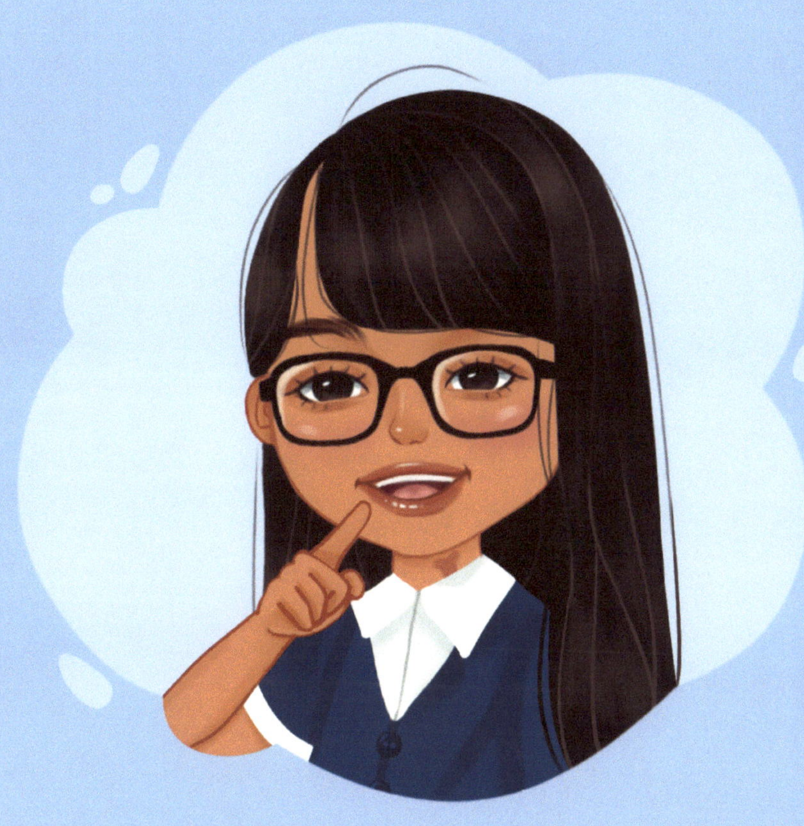

Exercise:

Try talking without using your tongue and see if others can understand you.

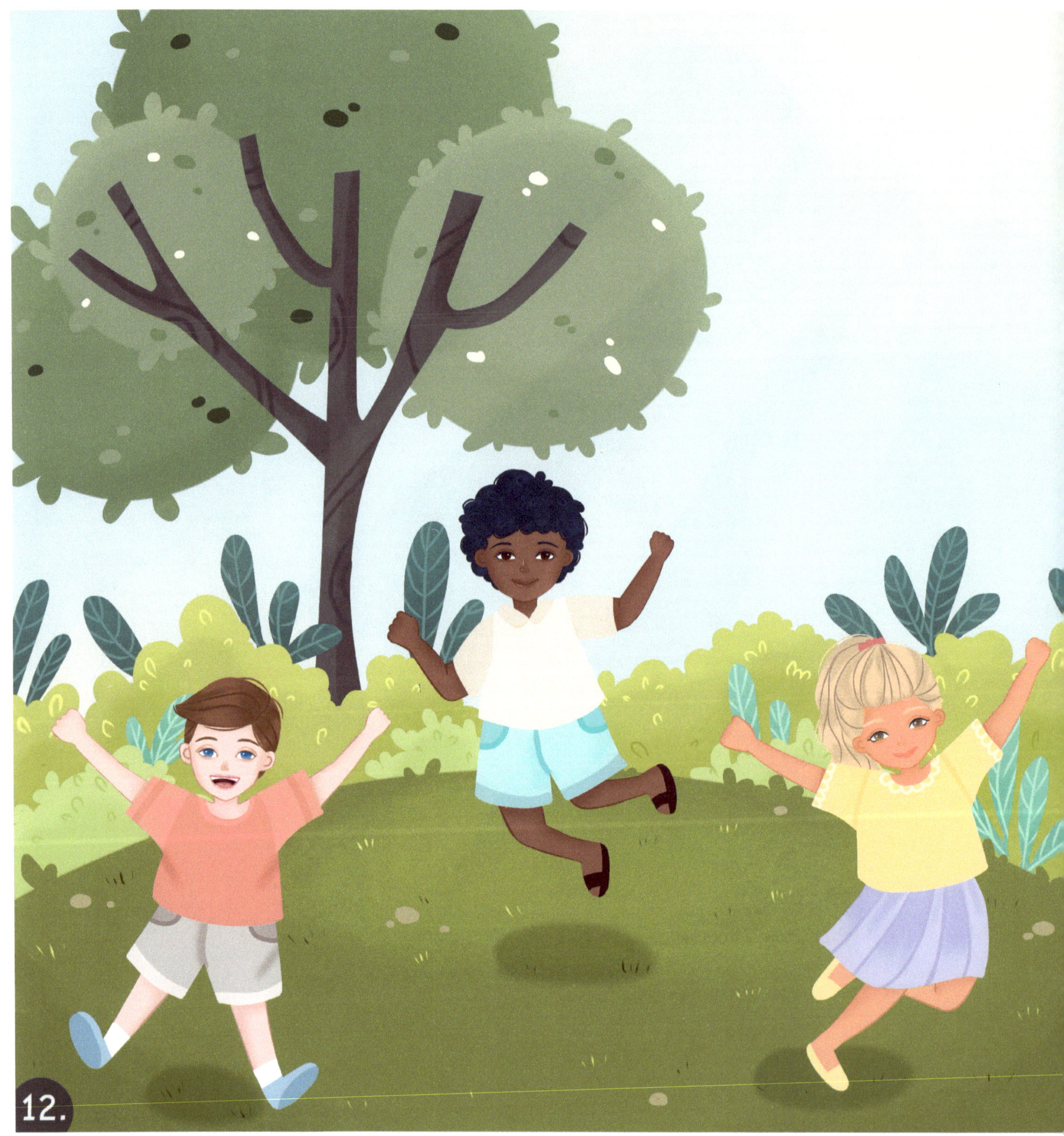

12.

Can you jump?

I can jump, but just a little. And it took me many hours of practice with my *physical therapist to be able to do it. You see, my muscles aren't as strong as they should be for my age. But it's okay, we are not competing; we are only having fun!

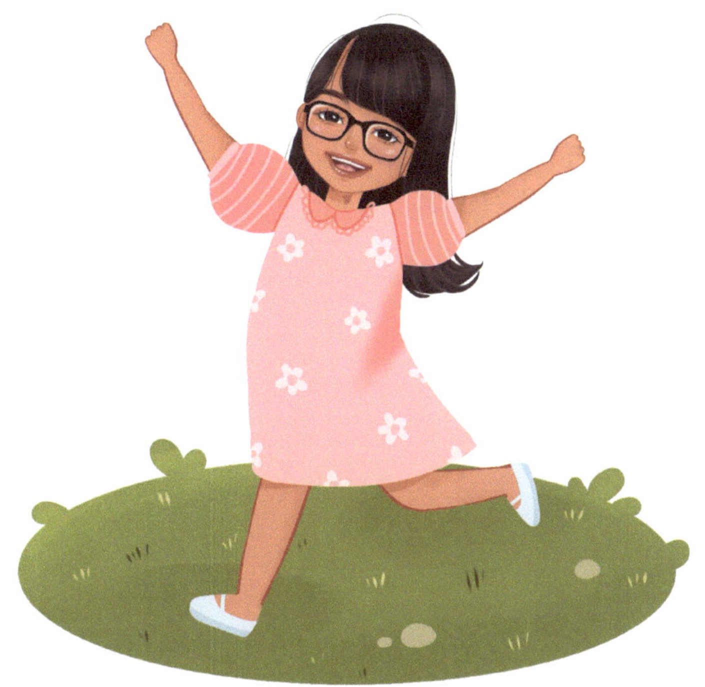

Can you ride a bicycle?

I can't, I have problems coordinating my movements and balancing when I am on a bicycle. Remember that all NF patients are unique, and some may have problems with learning how to ride a bicycle and others may not. But it's okay, I can do so many other things!

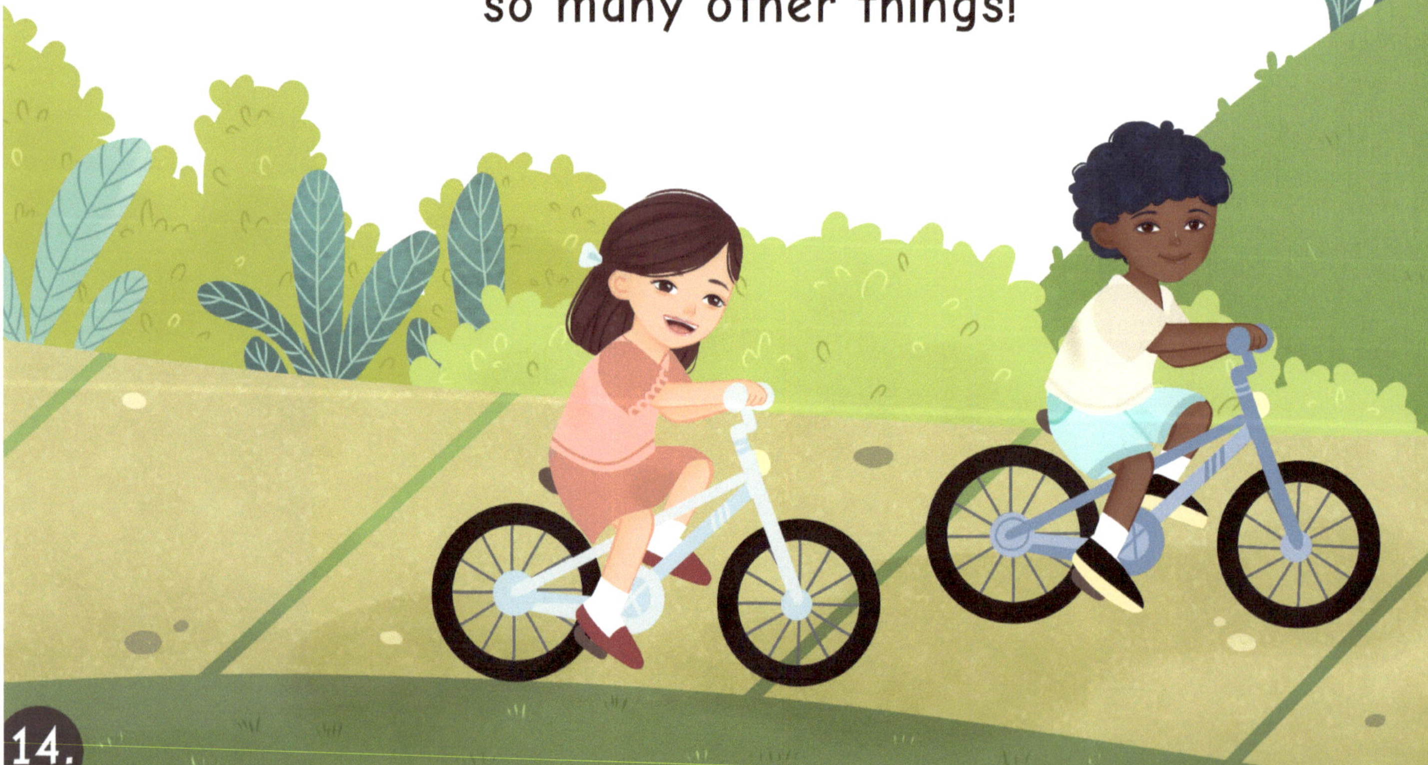

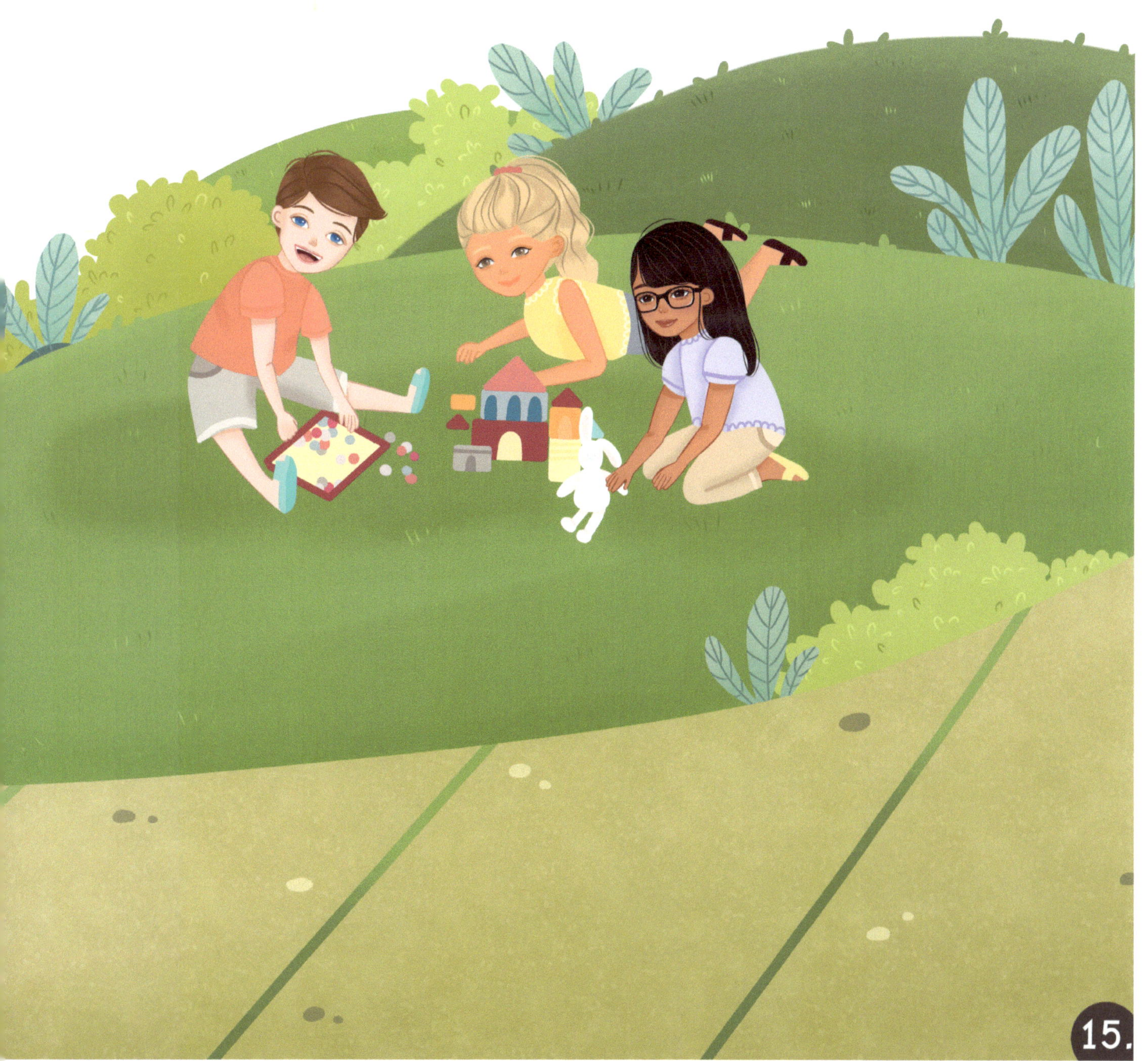

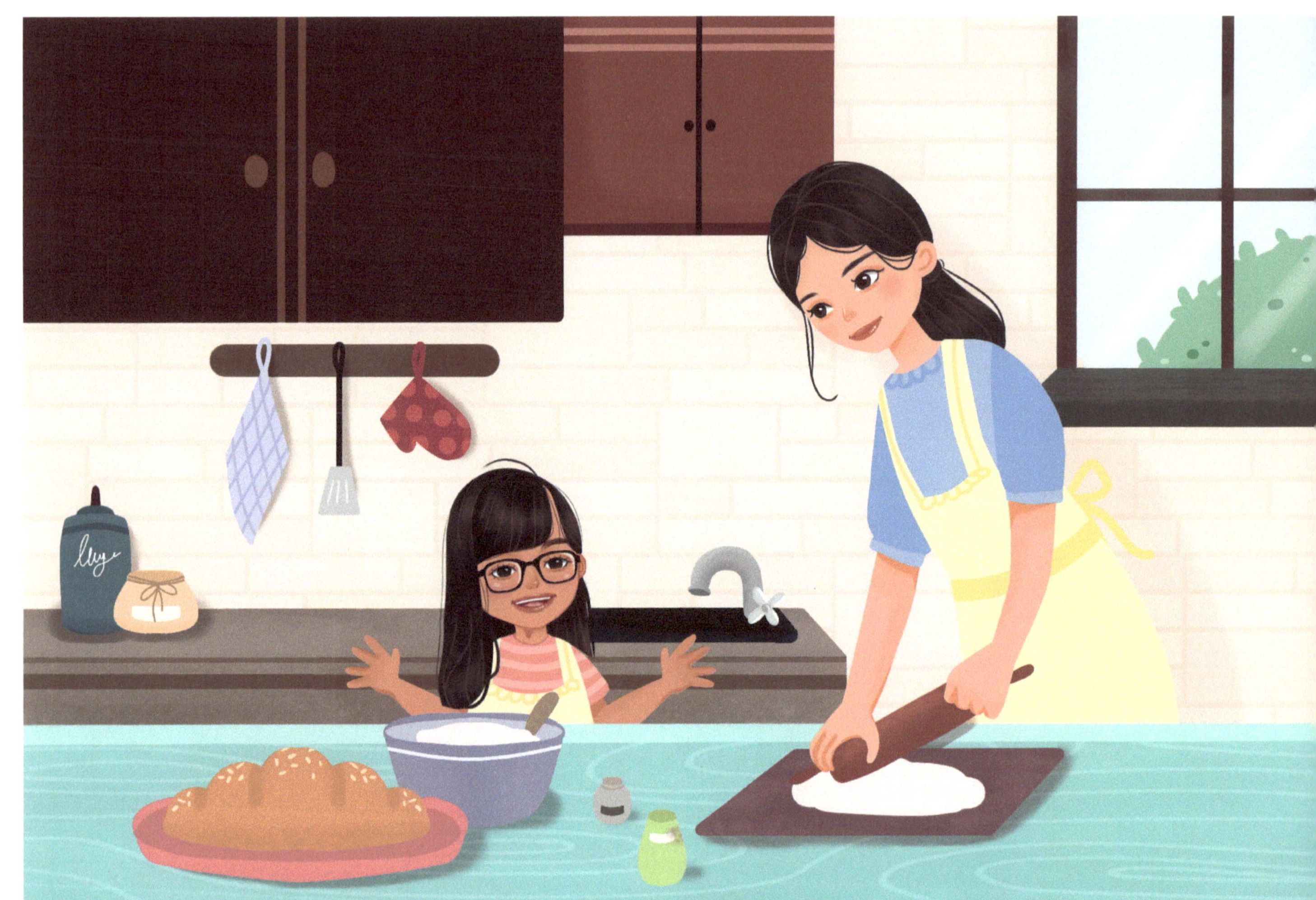

I can dance, I can paint, I can crochet, I practice karate, and I also like to bake. I learned to do all these things with my mom's help.

What things do you like to do for fun?

Exercise:

Share things you like to do for fun. Let's identify what you may have in common with other children.

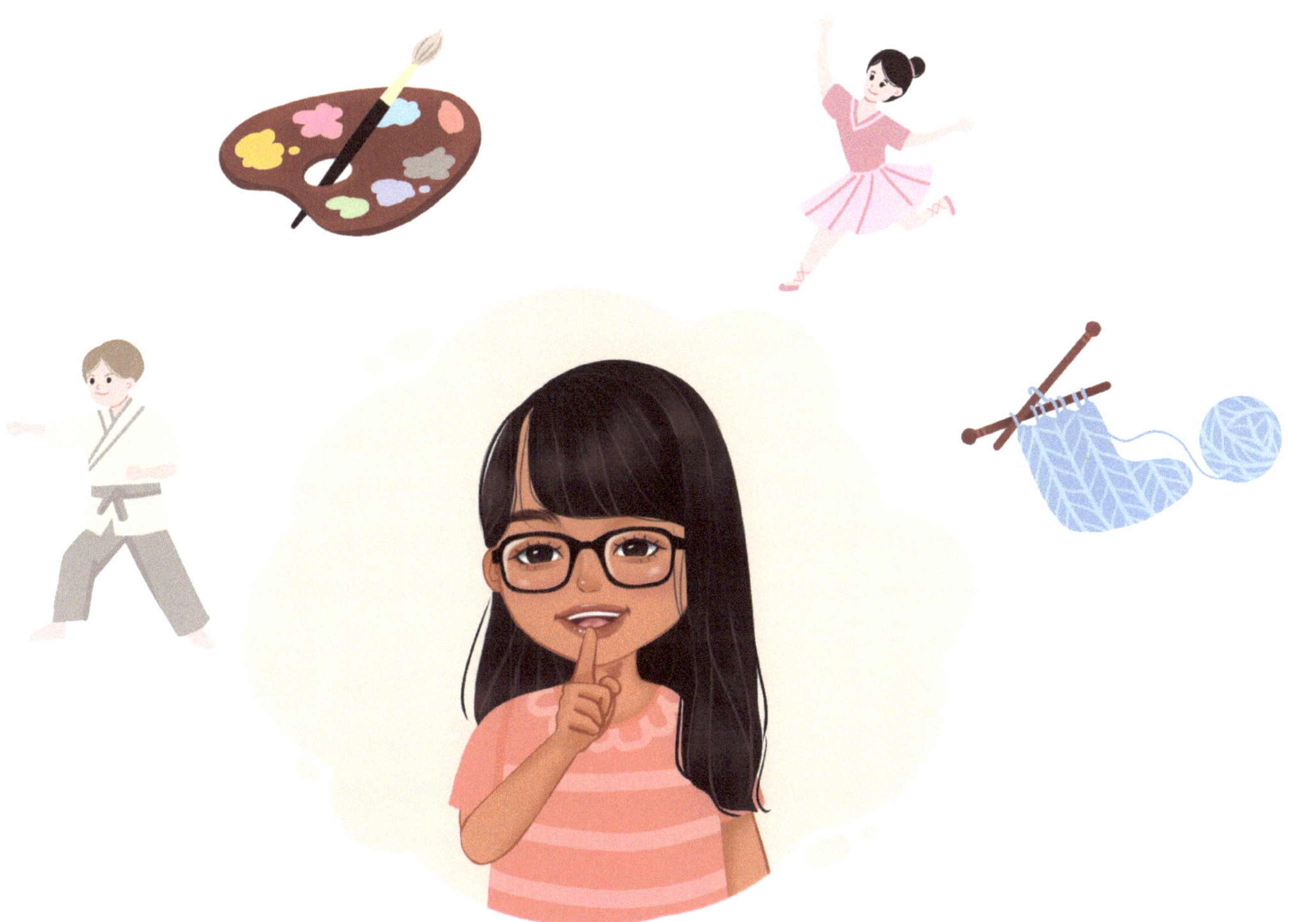

Why can't you see well?

Because of my muscle weakness, my eyes have also weakened. My left eye does not work well nor aligns with my right eye; this is known as *strabismus.

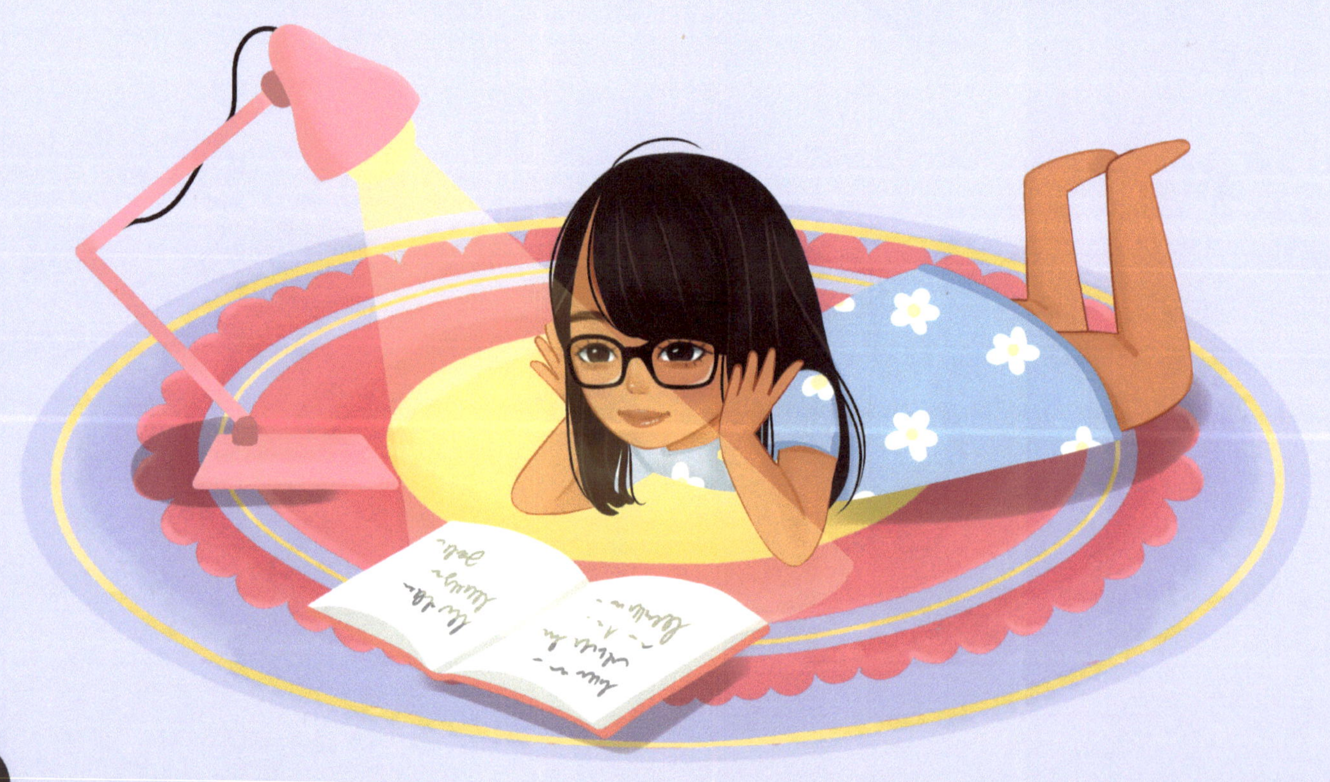

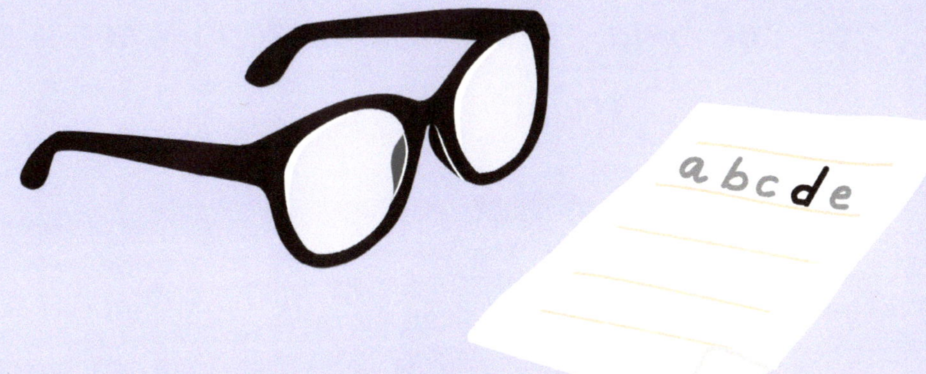

Exercise:

You can use plastic eyeglasses with blurry lenses, ask the reader to find a word or a letter to read out loud and let them share their experience with little visibility.

Oh wow! This was a lot of information, right?

Now you have the power of knowledge.

Therefore, you can help others understand what it's like to have NF.

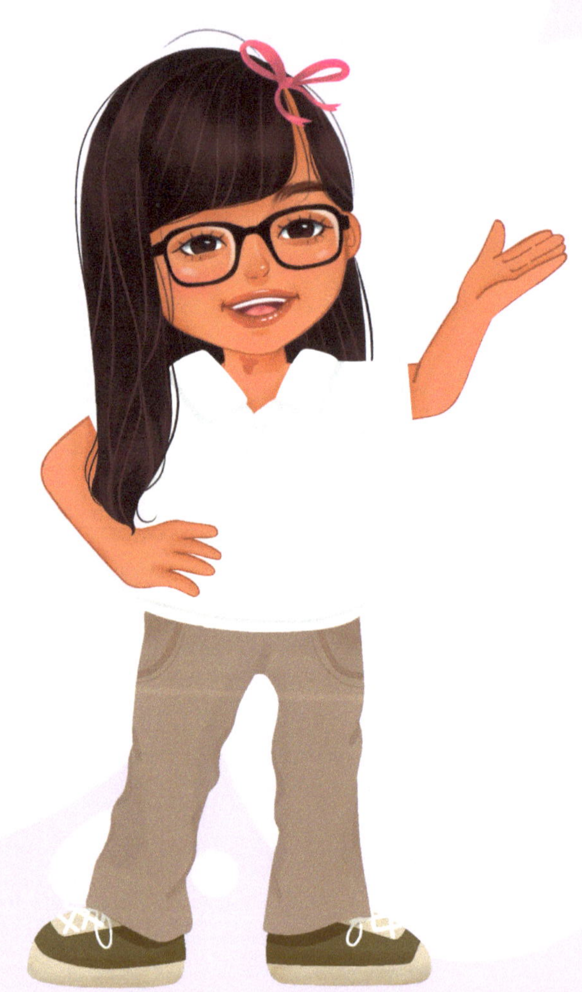

Thank you for reading this book and for joining us in this educational world of NF. As you have read, NF can cause many difficulties to a patient, including learning delays.

I appreciate you taking your time to understand what some children and adults with NF go through as they grow up in a world where they may not have the same opportunities as the general population because of how they look, speak, or behave.

As you may see there is so much more to having "café-au-lait" spots and tumors/neurofibroma in the NF community. Kindness comes a long way; and it can change the world.

It starts with you!

GLOSSARY

Café-au-lait: Café au lait spots, or café au lait macules, are flat, hyperpigmented birthmarks The name café au lait is French for "coffee with milk" and refers to their light-brown color. In contrast, café au lait lesions of neurofibromatosis have smooth borders.
They are caused by a collection of pigment-producing melanocytes in the epidermis of the skin.
These spots are typically permanent and may grow or increase in number over time.

Contagious: Something transmissible by contact.

Genetic condition: A genetic condition occurs when you inherit an altered (changed) gene from your parents that increases your risk of developing a particular condition. However not all genetic conditions are passed down from your parents, some gene changes occur randomly before you are born.

Hypotonia: Hypotonia means decreased muscle tone.

Inherited: - occurring among members of a family usually by heredity; "an inherited disease"; "familial traits"; "genetically transmitted features"

Nervous system: The organized network of nerve tissue in the body. It includes the central nervous system (the brain and spinal cord), the peripheral nervous system (nerves that extend from the spinal cord to the rest of the body), and other nerve tissue.

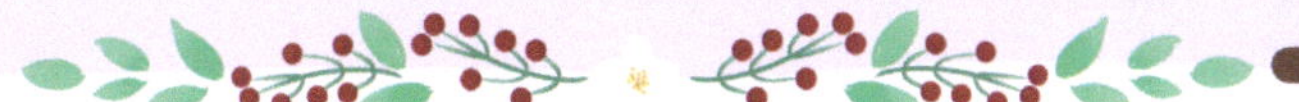

Neurofibromatosis: Neurofibromatosis is a genetic disorder of the nervous system. It mainly affects how nerve cells form and grow. It causes tumors to grow on nerves. You can get neurofibromatosis from your parents, or it can happen because of a mutation (change) in your genes. Once you have it, you can pass it along to your children. Usually the tumors are benign, but sometimes they can become cancerous.

There are three types of neurofibromatosis:

- Type 1 (NF1) causes skin changes and deformed bones. It usually starts in childhood. Sometimes the symptoms are present at birth.
- Type 2 (NF2) causes hearing loss, ringing in the ears, and poor balance. Symptoms often start in the teen years.
- Schwannomatosis causes intense pain. It is the rarest type.

Many health conditions run in families. Genetic conditions are often called hereditary because they can be passed from parents to their children.

Physical therapist: A health professional trained to evaluate and treat people who have conditions or injuries that limit their ability to move and do physical activities.

Spontaneous mutation: A spontaneous mutation of a gene belonging to a chromosome is one that occurs unexpectedly without having been inherited from the parents and can lead to a genetic disorder or disease.

Strabismus: is a disorder in which both eyes do not line up in the same direction. Therefore, they do not look at the same object at the same time. The most common form of strabismus is known as "crossed eyes."

Tumors/neurofibroma:
A benign tumor that develops from the cells and tissues that cover nerves.

Jamaly's picture and poem

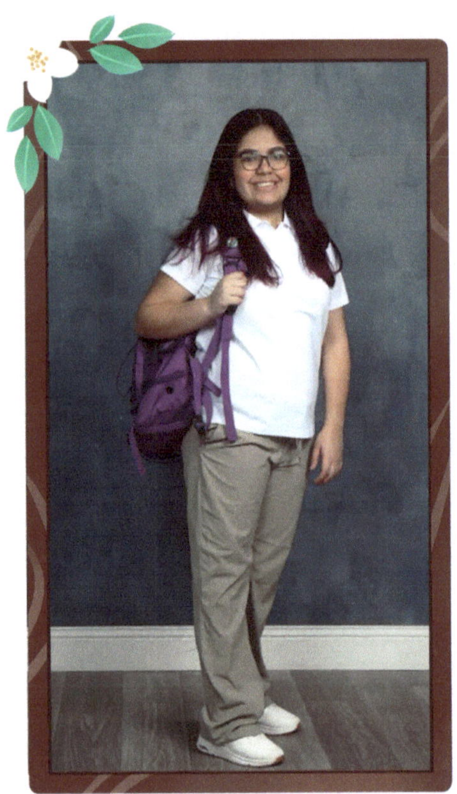

This is Who I Am

I am strong,
I am smart,
I am different,
I am hopeful, and
I am loved,
This is who I am,

I am joyful, and
I am sometimes in pain,
But I have love,
This is who I am.

I am a fighter,
I am resilient, and
I will win this battle,
This is who I am.

If you want to learn more about Neurofibromatosis (NF), there are so many nonprofit organizations and resources that will help you understand and help children like Jamy. Please see information below. You will find different websites with more information about NF.

Resource websites

-Neurofibromatosis | NF | MedlinePlus (english)
https://medlineplus.gov/neurofibromatosis.html

-Genetic conditions
(https://www.healthywa.wa.gov.au/Articles/F_I/Genetic-conditions)

 •NCI Search Results - NCI (cancer.gov) (English)
 https://www.cancer.gov/search/results?swKeyword=neurofibroma

 •NCI Search Results - NCI (cancer.gov) (English)
 https://www.cancer.gov/search/results?swKeyword=Nervous+system

-Café au lait spot - (English)
https://dermnetnz.org/topics/cafe-au-lait-macule

-Hypotonia: MedlinePlus Medical Encyclopedia (English)
https://medlineplus.gov/ency/article/003298.htm

-NCI Search Results - NCI (cancer.gov) (English)
https://www.cancer.gov/search/results?swKeyword=Physical+therapist

-Strabismus: MedlinePlus Medical Encyclopedia (English)
https://medlineplus.gov/ency/article/001004.htm